The China Study ...in 30 minutes

D1453470

THE EXPERT GUIDE TO **T. COLIN CAMPBELL'S**

The China Study

...in 30 minutes

THE 30 MINUTE EXPERT SERIES

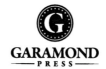

GARAMOND
— PRESS —

A NOTE TO THE READER: You should purchase and read the book that has been reviewed. This book is meant to accompany a reading of the reviewed book and is neither intended nor offered as a substitute for the reviewed book.

This review is unofficial and unauthorized. This book is not authorized, approved, licensed, or endorsed by T. Colin Campbell, PhD, Thomas M. Campbell II, or BenBella Books.

Contents

At a Glance

This book is an abridged overview of *The China Study*, a best seller focusing on the relationship between nutrition and disease. The authors, a father-and-son team—T. Colin Campbell, PhD, and Thomas M. Campbell II, MD—describe in great detail a major study conducted in China that began in 1982 and continues today. The study is a collaboration between the authors and Chinese scientists, and it received the approval of both the Chinese and US governments. While observational studies of humans are being conducted in China, animal research studies are being performed in the United States. The data from the research and study are important to the authors' conclusions and are summarized in the book.

This overview provides a brief introduction to *The China Study*, and then moves on to cover information regarding both the book and the authors. As part of the analysis of the importance of this book, this review includes a brief rundown of readers' responses (both positive and negative), from professional reviewers as well as readers from the general public, followed by a synopsis of *The China Study*. The next section discusses the three main concepts of the book, including examples and ideas of how these concepts can be applied to you. Finally, the main points are restated, in a way that will perhaps convince you to get a copy of the book and see for yourself the remarkable research done and the conclusions drawn by these eminent scientists. Also included is a list of key terms, along with their definitions, and a related reading list, with a brief description of each book.

Understanding
The China Study

ABOUT THE BOOK

With the title *The China Study: The Most Comprehensive Study of Nutrition Ever Conducted and the Startling Implications For Diet, Weight Loss, and Long-Term Health,* it might seem like this book is overreaching. However, this is not an exaggeration; the scope of the research and related studies is unprecedented. The authors studied 6,500 adults from various counties and provinces in China, analyzing their diet and health and reaching stunning conclusions about the direct relationship between nutrients and several diseases, such as cancer, diabetes, heart failure, and other lethal ailments plaguing the Western world.

The book sheds light on those afflictions and the direct link between them and the consumption of protein from an animal-based diet. This connection was first discovered in a study in India, which showed that ingested animal protein had a clear link to liver cancer. The authors paid particular attention to the impact of animal-based proteins on human health. The conclusion of that exhaustive study is that a vegan (no animal-based foods) diet is the healthiest way to eat. Plants provide all the nutrients the human body needs to function properly and to fend off disease. Meat, milk, and other dairy products have been linked to liver cancer in many of the Chinese subjects of the study. For Westerners who grew up thinking that cow's milk is the perfect food, these conclusions are revolutionary, and call for a drastic change in lifestyle and food consumption. The China Study is still ongoing, thirty-five years after it started.

Although it was written by scientists, *The China Study* delivers practical information and research findings in accessible language with the layperson in mind. The book includes personal anecdotes, and the authors are at times humorous in their approach. The authors feel strongly about their mission to inform the public about a range of issues, including the causes of disease and the impact of special-interest groups on public understanding. The book contains dozens of graphs and charts illustrating the conclusions of the scientists who conducted this and related studies. The information in these diagrams supplements the narrative and supports the authors' assertions through various case studies.

ABOUT THE AUTHORS

T. Colin Campbell, a highly regarded nutrition scientist, was born in 1934 and raised on a dairy farm, where he helped care for the animals and milk the cows. His mother had a large garden, and they produced most of the food they ate. As was typical at that time, their diet was heavily weighted toward animal protein, supplemented by garden vegetables.

Campbell attended Pennsylvania State University for three years, majoring in pre-veterinary medicine. He received early admission to the University of Georgia School of Veterinary Medicine, which he attended for one year. At that point, he received an unsolicited offer of a scholarship to do graduate research in animal nutrition and the relatively new field of biochemistry at Cornell University. He received his master's degree in 1957 and went on to work as a technician at an animal research lab, testing various chemicals and irradiated foods to see if they would cause cancer in animals. It was at this point that he became involved in what ultimately would become his life's work—the effects of nutrition on health.

In 1959, also at Cornell, Campbell began working toward his PhD in animal nutrition, with minors in biochemistry and microbiology, and he presented his dissertation in 1961. He was offered a position in a new toxicology laboratory at the Massachusetts Institute of Technology (MIT) in 1963, where he continued his research into toxins, especially those considered to be carcinogenic. In 1965 he moved to Virginia Tech as a lecturer in biochemistry and toxicology. He also continued his research, working as the coordinator of a US State Department project in the Philippines that focused on developing feeding centers for malnourished children—a project that pointed to the negative results of a protein-based diet. He was also a member of the National Academy of Sciences and sat on various panels examining the effects of saccharin as used in food and drinks.

In 1975, Campbell returned to Cornell as a full professor, where he continued his experimental research until 1996. The Campbell research lab hosted a visiting Chinese scholar for a year in 1980, and Campbell was introduced to the observational research related to nutrition that was just beginning in China. The US government's National Institutes of Health (NIH) and the government of China were persuaded to fund and begin observational studies in China that would also relate to the animal nutritional research studies being conducted in the United States. So began the years-long project, still in progress today, that has come to be known as the China Study, the most comprehensive study of health and nutrition ever conducted.

Campbell has authored or coauthored over 350 scientific papers published in the most prestigious scientific journals, has testified before numerous congressional committees and subcommittees, and has traveled the world giving hundreds of speeches and presentations regarding the relationship between nutrition and disease. He is currently collaborating with his son, Thomas M. Campbell II, on continuing studies and public education concerning nutrition and its effects on public health. He lives in Ithaca, NY, with his wife, Karen.

Thomas M. Campbell II, is a 1999 graduate of Cornell University. He is currently pursuing a medical career after receiving his MD in 2010, and his practice emphasizes lifestyle medicine and health promotion. He often collaborates with his father and gives presentations regarding health and nutrition.

CRITICAL RECEPTION

The Upside

Although published in 2005 by BenBella Books, a small publisher in Texas, *The China Study* has gone on to sell over five hundred thousand copies and is still selling strongly today. In multiple interviews, former US president Bill Clinton has talked about his nutritional conversion from fast-food carnivore to vegan following two heart surgeries, citing *The China Study* and Dean Ornish as primary motivators and sources of his lifestyle change. Ornish, a physician and author of several well-received books about nutrition and heart disease, states that *"The China Study* is one of the most important books about nutrition ever written—reading it may save your life." Likewise, Joel Fuhrman, author of the popular book *Eat to Live*, calls *The China Study* "a fascinating read ... that could change the future for all of us. Every health care provider and researcher in the world must read it."

A review in *Independent Science News* said that *"The China Study* excels at clear explanations and data-based reasoning that together inform but also challenge scientists and nonscientists to rethink current scientific and dietary assumptions." Many reactions from general readers on bookseller websites are positive and range from referring to the book as "life-changing" and "amazing" to "should be required reading."

The Downside

Alongside controversy about the best dietary path human beings can take for optimal health, several researchers and fellow scientists have also taken the Campbells to task regarding their interpretation of various data and for generalizing the nutritional content of foods. Lawrence Wilson, who has both personal and professional interests in vegetarian and vegan diets, stated on his website, DrLWilson.com, that "This book is often cited

... as being a definitive study and guide to the superiority of vegetarianism. However, upon careful review of this book, it is no such thing." He goes on to list various common health problems associated with vegetarian and vegan diets, such as low levels of specific vitamins or minerals, and continues with a list of what he calls "factual errors." He suggests that "a much better book on this subject is by Weston Price, DDS, titled *Nutrition and Physical Degeneration.*"

In a review on *Raw Food SOS*, Denise Minger examined the data and concluded that the book was based on some serious flaws in reasoning, stating at one point that "when we actually track down the direct correlation between animal protein and cancer, there is no statistically significant positive trend. ... The only way Campbell could indict animal protein is by throwing a third variable—cholesterol—into the mix." The authors have responded to criticism of their data interpretation, scientific methodology, and conclusions with further explanation of biological plausibility and how it has helped to explain statistical correlations and inform their assumptions. Still, the controversy continues.

SYNOPSIS

Throughout his more than half century of laboratory research and observational studies on animals and humans, T. Colin Campbell has worked to show that nutrition has a direct bearing on health and disease. Having been born and raised on a farm, he, along with most Americans, thought that a healthful diet consisted of meat, eggs, dairy products, fruit, and vegetables. To this day, the Food and Drug Administration (FDA) Food Pyramid contains these items, along with nuts and grains.

However, beginning with his initial research in the 1950s studying the effects of certain toxins on the rates of liver cancer in mice, Campbell suspected that another culprit was at play. After working in the Philippines with malnourished children and children sick with liver cancer, and subsequently reading a scientific article from India detailing the effects of protein ingestion on liver cancer in mice, he began to gain insights. Although Campbell worked at several different labs during his career, he always pursued the idea that nutrition has a direct bearing on overall human health and the disease processes that are the most frequent causes of death in the United States.

After the easing of political tensions between China and the United States, Campbell was introduced to the observational comparative studies of the incidence of cancer that were taking place in China. His professional acquaintance with a high-ranking Chinese health official, along with his sterling reputation in the scientific arena, prompted the unusual cooperation of the US government's National Institutes of Health (NIH) and the Chinese government in a joint observational and comparative study that has been expanded and continues to this day. The research has come to be known as the China Study.

The project started with an atlas of China that showed that there were substantial variations in both the incidence and the types of cancer, depending on geographic location. The questions immediately raised were about environmental and lifestyle effects on various cancers, since most Chinese people are genetically homogenous. The original "cancer atlas" included the incidences of over four dozen diseases, including individual cancers, heart disease, and infectious diseases. The research team visited sixty-five rural counties and administered questionnaires, took blood and urine samples from over 6,500 adults, directly measured everything eaten by the study subjects over a three-day period, and analyzed food samples from local markets. After the numbers were crunched, the results were remarkable.

In the United States, about 15 percent of the calories that people consume come from animal protein. The rural Chinese, on the other hand, consume a diet with only 9 or 10 percent of calories derived from animal protein, with most food sources being plant-based. These findings directly correlated with the types and incidences of diseases suffered by Americans and the Chinese. Those whose proteins were derived from plants were more likely to die from diseases of nutritional inadequacy and poor sanitation, such as digestive or parasitic diseases, while those who consumed protein from animal sources succumbed mostly to diseases associated with "nutritional extravagance," such as cancer, diabetes, and heart disease.

These observations were supported by clinical animal research studies, which also showed that various disease processes could be stopped or even reversed by reducing the amount of protein in the diet and by ensuring that the protein sources were plants rather than animals. The implications were staggering. What the China Study showed is that most disease processes that afflict Americans and other Westernized societies can be slowed down, made dormant, or avoided entirely, merely by implementing nutritional changes. By eliminating animal-based protein and turning to plants as the primary source of food, health and wellness can be dramatically improved and many frightening diseases avoided altogether.

Key Concepts of
The China Study

According to the Campbells, Americans are experiencing a health care crisis of immense proportions due in no small part to the unwittingly combined efforts of the **food industries, science, medicine, and the government**. In the book, they examine the results of the China Study, comparing **Eastern versus Western nutrition and disease** rates. Additionally, they look at nutrition as it relates to the most common chronic diseases suffered by Americans today and conclude that, indeed, **you are what you eat**.

I. FOOD INDUSTRIES, SCIENCE, MEDICINE, AND THE GOVERNMENT

Nearly 2,500 years ago, the Greek philosopher Plato wrote that societies living in luxury were destined for sickness and disease. Hippocrates, the father of Western medicine, fervently advocated lifestyle changes for improved health. In the nineteenth century, George Macilwain wrote fourteen books about the subject and applied his findings to the diet of his family and patients. Researchers and scientists have studied the correlation between food and health since the early twentieth century. In the past four decades, many prominent physicians, including Caldwell Esselstyn, Dean Ornish, and John McDougall, have studied plant-based diets and integrated them into their practices. Today, it is widely accepted in scientific circles that avoiding animal-based foods and embracing a whole-food, plant-based diet staves off or even cures chronic life-threatening diseases while promoting robust health.

With over 80 percent of the American population at high risk for chronic diseases such as heart disease, cancer, or diabetes, this information should be more widely available to the public, taught in schools, and imparted during every visit to the family doctor. With documented positive correlations between plant-based diets and lower rates of disease as well as weight loss, why is the general public not more educated and informed regarding nutrition and its effect on chronic diseases?

There are a number of reasons, but mostly it comes down to greed and self-interest. As the authors state, much of the medical and research industry is governed by the golden rule: he who has the gold makes the rules. There is a vast amount of money to be made from pharmaceuticals that address "diseases of affluence," with conservative estimates as high as $1 trillion per year. As any good businessperson would say, these enterprises must do everything they can to protect and increase their profits. The entire system, including industries related to health care, food production, government, science, and medicine, seems to promote profits over health. The system may or may not be overtly corrupt, but it is certainly incestuous, with various entities overlapping and many times becoming indistinguishable from one another in their quest to advance their own interests over the public good.

The problem begins with the food industry. Plant-based food products are not as profitable as animal-based products. Therein lies the reason for all the organizations and lobbying groups that represent the animal-based food industry: the National Dairy Council, American Meat Institute, National Cattlemen's Association, National Livestock and Meat Board, National Pork Producers Council, and United Egg Producers, to name just a few. These lobbying organizations exist to do nothing more than promote their products. Some efforts are quite transparent—for example, print ads and billboards. Others are rather insidious, like providing public schools with tools and study plans that supposedly teach good nutrition but in reality promote the consumption of meat and dairy products over fruits and vegetables.

The food industry also provides funding for research studies regarding the effects of various chemical compounds and nutrients found in various food sources. On the surface, this sounds quite altruistic, but what the food industry is looking for is a "hook": something they can use to convince consumers to purchase more of their product. For instance, when it was discovered that conjugated linoleic acid (CLA), which is produced in cows and excreted in milk, had an inhibitory effect on the formation of stomach tumors in mice, the National Dairy Council, which had funded the research, started to release information and press packets indicating that drinking more milk could fight cancer.

The discovery of CLA also highlights one of the problems in the science arena. Funding issues promote an environment where researchers are more inclined to investigate the effects of certain chemicals or individual nutrients on health and disease rather than focusing on overall nutrition, a practice that the authors call "scientific reductionism." For example, a few years ago, it was discovered that lycopene, a carotenoid that causes the red coloration in tomatoes, was shown to reduce the incidence of prostate cancer in laboratory animals. A few (less than five) human studies appeared to back this up; however, the human subjects were not consuming isolated lycopene. They were consuming tomatoes and tomato products that contained lycopene, meaning that there could be other components or qualities in tomatoes that were causing the positive results. Nonetheless, the food and supplement industries hopped aboard the lycopene train, touting the cancer-preventing qualities of lycopene in an attempt to boost sales of their products. This kind of reductionism is as faulty as making generalizations.

Of course, many physicians and other health care professionals are too busy to read the research and make their own determinations. They also generally have not been properly trained in nutrition or prevention, leaving them with the "knowledge" that drugs and surgery are the answers to chronic diseases. For updates on new research findings, they rely on information gleaned from various media sources or distributed by pharmaceutical companies. Additionally, although many doctors acknowledge the positive effects of a healthful diet, they don't have the time to sit down with their patients and counsel them. Moreover, a large number of physicians—cardiologists, for example—have been taught since medical school primarily about physical intervention after the fact, such as inserting a stent after a heart attack, as opposed to educating patients about the prevention of heart disease through nutrition.

When advising patients, most physicians rely on government nutritional guidelines issued by the FDA, which have been heavily influenced by the animal-based food-product industries. For instance, although FDA recommendations include the statement that five daily servings of fruit or vegetables are a primary part of a healthful diet, they also allow up to 35 percent of daily calories to be composed of fat. The FDA also says that 45 percent of calories can be carbohydrates (with an upper limit of 25 percent of those carbohydrates being refined sugar products), and a whopping 35 percent can be derived from protein. Not only do these numbers not add up, they also confuse the public into thinking that consuming a high-fat, high-protein diet is healthful.

Government plays its part in this debacle as well. Although some research funding comes from the taxpayer, due to budgetary constraints the bulk of it comes from private industry. This leaves the door wide open for conflict-of-interest issues, or even outright abuse of research standards stemming from the ability of commercial interests to design the studies, choose the scientists, and "spin" the results so as to be seen in a positive light by the general public, all in an attempt to increase profits. The government is forced to rely on the results produced by private research, and in many cases, misinformation is fed to the public via government sources, leading people to believe what is being said, whether it is actual fact or "spun" information.

All in all, it is a vicious circle. Companies want to make profits. The public wants to be healthy. Government cannot fund all proposed nutritional research, so many scientists rely on the private sector for these funds. Agribusiness and pharmaceutical companies step in to fund research that helps to promote their products. Many of these studies are skewed or incomplete, but the results are fed to the media. Government officials are influenced by the powerful food-industry lobby, and they have traditionally caved in to pressures brought on them in regard to setting nutrition standards. Physicians are under-informed, and many rely on government organizations or pharmaceutical companies for their information. This has left Americans in a state of confusion, as it is nearly impossible to tell the difference between science and industry, government and science, or government and industry.

Examples from The China Study

- The National Dairy Council has worked diligently for almost one hundred years to promote dairy products, and it targets children more than any other demographic. The organization introduced "nutritional education" programs into public schools. Its website clearly states that the purpose of the council (renamed Dairy Management Inc. in 1995) is to promote and market milk and other dairy products through schools, partnerships with major food marketers like Kraft and Kellogg's, and through government assistance platforms, especially the Special Supplemental Nutrition Program for Women, Infants, and Children (WIC). Their school programs are designed to teach children to become lifelong consumers of dairy products, as evidenced by two of their many "nutrition education" kits offered to elementary schools, "Pyramid Café" and "Pyramid Explorations." These kits include lesson plans, videos, posters, and teaching guides designed to assist teachers with the nutrition portion of their curriculum, while at the same time heavily promoting milk and other dairy products.

- Drug companies and medical practitioners have long shared a happy relationship. Health care professionals, especially physicians, are overworked and overwhelmed, giving them very little time to familiarize themselves with current research and new drug therapies. The pharmaceutical industry has stepped into this information vacuum, and today, most doctors receive new information regarding diseases and various therapies by reading the occasional article or from drug company representatives. Stocking a "sample cabinet" in the doctor's clinic is just one way that pharmaceutical industry reps introduce doctors to their product and increase sales. Although there are no kickbacks or other illegal activities, doctors sometimes attend drug company–sponsored seminars, often held in vacation spots, with all expenses paid for by the companies. Every health care professional is required to earn a certain number of Continuing Medical Education (CME) credits per year, and this requirement can be met by attending one or more events funded by the drug companies. While CME programs are overseen by US regulatory agencies, and the stated intention of these programs is to bring together medical professionals to increase awareness of certain issues or to further their research, many of the topics covered relate directly to new drugs being marketed by the companies.

Applying the Concept

- **Be skeptical.** You've undoubtedly heard the phrase, "If it sounds too good to be true, it probably is." Keep this in mind when you see or hear media reports regarding new drugs or fantastic cures. Question your doctor if he or she prescribes a new medication. Do your own research on it. Remember that drug companies have both the funds and the power to design research studies to fit their own agenda, which is ultimately to protect and increase their profits, not to protect your health.

- **Take USDA guidelines with a grain of salt.** As the authors point out, the FDA is heavily influenced by both the pharmaceutical and the food lobbies. Even though there are now hundreds of studies that show the positive impact of a plant-based diet that contains low levels of protein, fats, and refined carbohydrates, the new nutrition guidelines released by the FDA a few years ago directly contradict the results presented by these studies. As suggested, keep your protein intake to about 10 percent of your total calorie intake, and limit your fat consumption to around 20 percent, making sure that the fat is not of the saturated variety. Limit your refined carbohydrates, opting instead for whole grains, fruit, and vegetables rather than white bread, white rice, or pastries.

- **Educate yourself.** With all the hype and promises of new "miracle" cures, and with conflicting information coming out regarding what constitutes proper nutrition, it is best to educate yourself rather than relying on the media and advertising. Refer to the Recommended Reading section to start your quest for better health and weight loss.

II. EASTERN VERSUS WESTERN NUTRITION AND DISEASE

At the outset of his landmark scientific analysis of the impact of nutrition on the course of various diseases, T. Colin Campbell was able to take advantage of opportunities that arose when tensions between China and the United States eased in the late 1970s. Science, politics, and financing all came together for an opportunity to finally observe the effects of nutrition and diet on a large, mostly homogenous human population, namely, the Chinese.

Campbell was first introduced to what would ultimately become known as the China Study when a distinguished visiting Chinese scientist showed him a color-coded atlas of China that showed the incidence of various cancers broken down by county. The atlas clearly showed that different cancers were geographically localized. Because the Chinese are genetically relatively homogenous—87 percent of the Chinese population is of Han ancestry—the incidence of these cancers could be explained by environmental causes. The map virtually begged the researchers to examine several questions: Why was there such a vast difference in the incidence of cancer in different counties? Why was cancer so much less prevalent in China than in the United States? And to what factors could these cancers be attributed?

Originally, the Chinese study looked at various cancers, but it was quickly expanded to include other diseases, such as diabetes, heart disease, and infectious diseases. In all, the incidence of four dozen diseases was examined. The researchers participating in the joint project elected to conduct their studies in rural areas due to the fact that rural people historically remained in the same county where they were born and ingested the same type of diet for their entire lives. A total of 6,500 adult villagers from over 170 villages in sixty-five rural and semirural counties were given a questionnaire and asked for blood and urine samples. Everything they ate over a three-day period was analyzed, as was the food available from local markets.

The results were remarkable. The research team ultimately found over eight thousand statistically significant associations among diet, lifestyle, and the incidence of various diseases, including cancer. Corresponding animal studies were also able to shed light on the effects of nutrition on the disease processes themselves. Combined, the information obtained from the Chinese observational studies and results from the animal studies done in the United States and elsewhere showed overwhelming correlations between diet and disease.

In the United States, about 15 percent of the average diet consists of protein. Of that protein, 80 percent is derived from animal products such as meat, dairy, fish, and eggs. In rural China, 9 to 10 percent of total calories ingested are protein, and only 10 percent of those calories come from animal sources. Additionally, the Chinese typically consumed around 2,600 calories per day, compared with the roughly 2,000 calories consumed per day by Americans, but the Chinese were rarely overweight. Conversely, Americans are in the middle of an obesity epidemic. These numbers suggest that there are major nutritional differences between the traditional American—or Western—diet and the traditional rural Chinese diet.

To further bolster these nutritional findings, the researchers looked at diets and disease in wealthier Chinese counties, although they did not perform the same comprehensive studies that they had done in the rural counties. Still, the results neatly complemented the conclusions drawn by the investigators—that diet and nutrition play a major and critical role in disease processes. They found that as people became more affluent, they tended to eat more animal products, and disease rates soared. It was determined that even those who relocated from rural areas to metropolitan areas had a higher incidence of heart disease, cancer, and other chronic illnesses after their relocation to the cities, confirming that environmental factors played a large role in the development and progress of these diseases in the population. These findings prompted the researchers to dub the chronic illnesses such as cardiovascular diseases, cancers, diabetes, and high cholesterol found in Westernized societies as "diseases of affluence" or "nutritional extravagance." The ailments that regularly occurred in rural areas, such as pneumonia, parasitic infestations, digestive diseases, and tuberculosis were categorized as "diseases of poverty."

After further assessment of the data, the research team concluded that one of the strongest predictors of Western diseases, diseases of affluence, is the level of blood cholesterol. Populations that consume animal products have far higher blood cholesterol levels than those consuming a plant-based diet. Much of the cholesterol found in the Western body is from dietary sources, and dietary cholesterol comes from animal-based foods. What the researchers found was that as the intake of dietary cholesterol increased, the incidence of Western diseases increased as well. Another surprise was that the Chinese who had "high" levels of blood cholesterol actually presented levels that were considered low by Western medical standards. Furthermore, as blood cholesterol levels decreased even more, down into the range rarely seen by Western physicians, so did the incidence of many cancers, including liver, colorectal, lung, breast, stomach, and esophageal, as well as the rate of leukemia. Additionally, the researchers found a correlation between low levels of cholesterol and extraordinarily low rates of heart disease, which is the number-one killer in Westernized societies.

Though he grew up on a farm and spent most of his adult life following FDA guidelines for optimal nutrition, consuming animal products as part of his daily diet regimen, Campbell was so convinced by the results of the China Study as well as the concurrent animal studies that he changed his diet and that of his family. Today, the Campbells eat a plant-based diet containing whole (unprocessed) foods, with minimal protein and cholesterol intake. Although Campbell specifically states that he does not identify himself as vegan, due to the fact that veganism has many restrictions regarding using animals for any purpose (such as leather), he does adhere to a vegan diet for health reasons. Unprocessed foods, whole grains, legumes, nuts, seeds, plant-based oils, all parts of plants, including roots, tubers, stems, leaves, and the fruits and vegetables produced by these plants, have become the mainstays of the Campbell family diet.

Campbell is not alone in his advocacy of the nutritional benefits of eating a plant-based diet. Dean Ornish, MD, now a household name, first came to the public's attention when he published his findings regarding nutrition and heart disease, stating that the consumption of a plant-based diet could not only slow the progress of heart disease but actually reverse and prevent it. Caldwell Esselstyn Jr., MD, also a highly respected physician, has published several books touting the disease-preventing properties of plant-based diets and the health benefits that can be expected when people eliminate animal-based products from their diets. These authors cite numerous respected scientific studies when presenting their theories, and they all literally put their money where their mouths are by shunning animal-based food products and consuming a plant-based diet. All remain in excellent health.

The investigatory studies continue through the present day, but the research scientists have been able to conclusively state that lower blood cholesterol levels are linked to lower rates of heart disease, cancer, and other Western diseases. The corollary to that statement is that higher cholesterol, which is linked to dietary cholesterol derived from animal products, is connected to higher rates of Western diseases. Ultimately, the research team has postulated that consuming a diet that resembles the rural Chinese diet (whole foods, plant-based, low protein) will lead to a decreased chance of developing or dying from the Western diseases of affluence.

Examples from The China Study

- Although there has been a movement in dietary circles promoting high-protein weight-loss programs (most notoriously, the Atkins Diet), Campbell suspected decades ago that protein levels had an effect on the rate of growth of liver tumors. He initially worked with laboratory rats, injecting them with small doses of aflatoxin, a potent carcinogen found in peanut mold, to observe its effects as a cause of liver cancer in humans. At about the same time, he read a scientific paper written by researchers in India regarding aflatoxin and liver cancer, which also added the variable of protein ingestion by the rats. Their results indicated that rats fed a diet low in protein showed little or no growth in their tumors, while rats fed a higher dose of protein displayed rapid tumor growth. Intrigued, Campbell set out to reproduce the results described, and he was also able to produce findings showing a correlation between protein ingestion and liver tumor growth. He expanded this research via his observational studies conducted in China, where he was able to show positive correlations between the amount of protein contained in various diets and the incidence of cancer, as well as a positive correlation between consumption of plant-based proteins and lower cancer rates.

- Westernized medicine currently defines high cholesterol as anything above 240 milligrams per deciliter of blood (mg/dL). A rate of 200–239 mg/dL is considered borderline high, and anything below 200 mg/dL is considered normal. However, the China Study revealed that the Chinese generally show blood cholesterol levels of 90–170 mg/dL, and sometimes even as low as 60–70 mg/dL. Thus, even the highest Chinese blood cholesterol level is well below the Western definition of normal, leading researchers to conclude that there is a definite positive correlation between higher blood cholesterol levels and the onset and progress of "diseases of affluence," such as coronary heart disease, various cancers, diabetes, stroke, Alzheimer's, and kidney disease. They also concluded that lower blood cholesterol levels, even levels considered by Western medicine to be dangerously low but that are frequently found in the Chinese population, have a positive correlation with a lower incidence, or even nonexistence, of the top killers of people in Westernized societies.

Applying the Concept

- **Eat whole foods.** In understanding the results of the China Study, it is evident that whole-food-based diets can improve health. These foods are unprocessed or unrefined, or have been refined or processed as little as possible before being consumed, and typically do not contain any added ingredients, such as salt or fats. Examples include unpolished grains, beans, fruits, and vegetables.

- **Lower protein and cholesterol intake.** Dietary cholesterol and animal protein are two of the biggest nutritional threats to optimal health. Since both dietary cholesterol and animal protein are derived from the same source, lowering protein and cholesterol intake can easily be achieved by eliminating animal-based food products from the diet.

- **Do away with meat and dairy.** Although nonhomogenized dairy products can be considered "whole" foods, dairy is an animal-based food product and should thus be avoided. There are many plant-based dairy substitutes that can be used in place of animal milk protein.

Plants also provide dietary fiber, which is critical to the maintenance of proper gastrointestinal function (thus fending off colorectal cancer). Plants also deliver all of the nutrients necessary to sustain a healthy life. Although Campbell does not advocate worrying about very small amounts of animal proteins that might appear in meals, he does suggest that you generally try to exclude even small amounts from your diet.

III. YOU ARE WHAT YOU EAT

If the old adage "you are what you eat" is true, many Westerners are composed of sugar and fat, and are suffering from diseases they can avoid. As *The China Study* and related research on humans and lab animals conclude, a diet consisting of animal protein and dairy products is severely harmful to humans. In fact, the authors point to animal-based foods as the major culprit in most of the killer diseases affecting Americans and others in the Western world: heart disease, different types of cancer, autoimmune diseases, diabetes (both types 1 and 2), obesity, and numerous others.

Far too often, patients suffering from these diseases defer to physicians' recommendations of surgery, expensive drugs, chemotherapy, radiation, and other harmful, invasive treatments. At times, these treatments are unavoidable, but as the China Study and related studies prove, most of these killer diseases can be avoided, even reversed, with the right diet—one that consists of whole, unprocessed, plant-based foods.

Heart disease is the result of various afflictions, such as high cholesterol, hypertension, diabetes, and obesity. Similarly, the onset of type 2 diabetes ("adult" diabetes) is the result of obesity and a diet high in carbohydrates and protein. In short, all these ailments are interlinked, and the culprit, not surprisingly, is a diet poor in nutrients and fiber, yet rich in fats and proteins.

One of the most curable types of cancer is that of the large bowel, also known as colorectal cancer. Early detection of this cancer leads to surgery (the colon is long enough that removal of an affected section doesn't interfere with proper digestion), and many patients live long, healthy lives afterward. But to avoid colorectal cancer, a diet rich in fiber is the simplest preventive measure. Fiber is found only in plant-based food. It is not a nutrient, and the body doesn't digest it. Instead, the fiber helps the digestive system by providing bulk (if taken with water) that makes the digested food move smoothly down the digestive tract. Most Westerners develop polyps in the colon as a result of a diet lacking in fiber. In most cases, these polyps are benign, but far too often they become malignant. If they go undetected, the tumors can slough off cancer cells that spread to adjacent organs, most often the liver, where they form new tumors and cause death.

Type 1 diabetes, also known as childhood-onset diabetes, is an autoimmune disease. The body's immune system attacks the pancreas, preventing the generation of insulin and resulting in a lifelong ordeal of insulin shots, amputations, blindness, kidney failure, and heart attacks. While most of the medical establishment agrees that type 1 diabetes is genetic and unavoidable, the authors claim that infants fed cow's milk instead of being nursed for at least three months are the most prone to develop this disease. The explanation is that the protein in cow's milk causes human bodies to develop antibodies that proceed to attack the pancreas (hence it is an "autoimmune" disease) and render it irreversibly useless. Type 2 diabetes is a disease afflicting people who consume a diet rich in animal-based foods. It's a "disease of affluence," as the authors refer to it, and twenty-five million Americans are suffering from it, compared with very low numbers of Chinese people living in rural areas and subsisting on a diet of mostly plant-based foods.

Obesity has been in the news quite often in the past couple of decades, as Americans—and medical practitioners—have become aware of the severity of this phenomenon. Two in three Americans are overweight, and one in three Americans is obese. To calculate whether one is overweight or obese, physicians and other health care professionals use a formula that establishes the body mass index (BMI), which is the proportion of body fat relative to the rest of the body. BMI = weight in kilograms/height in meters squared. A BMI of 30 or higher means the person is obese; those at 25 to 29.9 are classified as overweight.

While not a disease by itself, obesity is a medical condition that can lead to many—often lethal—diseases. It has reached plague levels in the United States and is most common among poor and working-class people, who tend to rely on cheap junk food for sustenance because they cannot afford to buy whole foods and may not have the time to cook for their families while working long hours for low wages. The number of obese children in the country is steadily rising, and efforts by public figures to encourage children to eat whole, plant-based foods are the beginning of a trend to educate families on the benefits of such a diet. However, since many US public schools have meals provided by fast-food chains such as McDonald's, and host vending machines that sell sodas and other high-sugar items, fighting childhood obesity is an uphill battle.

Obesity is positively linked to high cholesterol, hypertension, cardiovascular disease, diabetes, and several types of cancer, including colorectal, breast, and prostate. It's a lifestyle disease, and it's preventable, or reversible, with the right diet and exercise.

Not surprisingly, the level of obesity in China is low, except in major metropolitan areas, where poverty is rampant. The many recent migrants to the cities, who have long been part of an agrarian society, are switching to fast food and other sources of harmful diets.

Examples from **The China Study**

COLORECTAL CANCER DEATH RATE IN "MORE DEVELOPED" COUNTRIES AND "LESS DEVELOPED" COUNTRIES

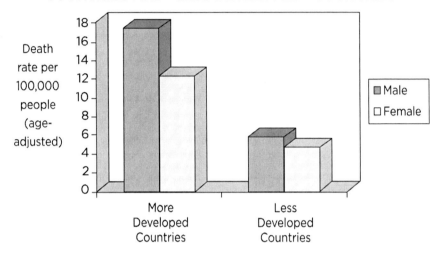

- The link between Western lifestyle and the high level of certain cancers, in this example colorectal cancer, is clear when compared to poorer countries, where meat and dairy aren't readily available and fiber-rich plant foods are dietary staples.

- James Anderson, MD, has been studying the effects of a high-fiber, low-fat, plant-based diet on fifty of his patients suffering from type 1 and type 2 diabetes. The results are nothing short of stunning. Although type 1 diabetes is incurable, Anderson's patients reduced their insulin intake by 30 percent after just three weeks. All but one of the type 2 patients discontinued their insulin intake altogether within weeks.

Applying the Concept

- **Calculate your BMI.** Using the formula provided earlier in this chapter, (or visit http://www.nhlbi.nih.gov/guidelines/obesity/BMI/bmicalc.htm), find out the fat level in your body compared to your total weight. If your BMI is 30 or higher, you're obese and can take immediate steps to lower your weight by switching to a whole-food, high-fiber, plant-based diet combined with exercise. Doing so, you'll be able to stop missing the enjoyable things in life and increase the limits on your mobility, mental health, self-perception, and social life. Understand that keeping weight off is a long-term endeavor and a lifestyle choice.

- **Don't give cow's milk to infants.** Although the medical establishment considers type 1 diabetes a genetic, unavoidable disease, the authors show a positive correlation between the consumption of cow's milk by infants and this devastating lifelong disease. At the very least, newborns should be nursed for three months so they can develop their immune system, thus fending off the harmful effects of cow's milk.

- **Genes aren't a death sentence.** Diseases proved to be linked to a genetic cause, such as breast cancer, colorectal cancer, and type 1 diabetes, aren't as big of a risk if you take dietary measures to prevent them, exercise, and are vigilant about screening for early detection of those cancers.

Key Takeaways

- In a perfect storm of competing interests, the food industries, science, medicine, and government have been drawn together to form the main sources of information regarding health and nutrition. Unfortunately, this combination has not worked well due to the fact that each group ultimately has its own goals, and the loser is likely to be the American public. With pharmaceutical companies "educating" physicians, the food industry "educating" children, and special-interest groups influencing entities like the World Health Organization for profit, improper nutrition in the United States is rapidly turning into a major health care crisis.

- Campbell and Campbell have shown, through exhaustive research of case studies, observational studies, and animal research studies, that consumption of animal protein and fat not only puts on unwanted pounds, but is a major factor in the development and progression of heart disease, cancer, diabetes, and a host of other "diseases of affluence" common in Westernized countries. They also show that the traditional diet found in China and other Eastern countries not only inhibits disease processes but may well prevent certain diseases.

- There is truth in the phrase "you are what you eat." Most people in industrialized nations consume diets high in saturated fats, refined sugars, processed grains, and chemically treated or genetically modified foods, leading to an epidemic of obesity and many chronic diseases that will ultimately kill. People in developing nations that consume a diet low in saturated fats, with few or no processed foods, generally don't eat themselves to death. Instead, they tend to suffer from other illnesses, such as tuberculosis and parasitic infestations.

A Final Word

A diet consisting of animal-based foods has definitively been proven to be linked to various diseases and other conditions by reputable scientists the world over. The myth of meat and milk as healthful (even "perfect") foods has been dispelled. For greater health and for weight loss, a plant-based diet, high in fiber and low in fat, is the answer. Humans can get all the nutrients they need from fruits, vegetables, whole grains, seeds, and nuts. Meat and dairy, contrary to widespread belief, are not the only source of protein and nutrients such as iron. In fact, protein and fat from plant-based foods are much healthier than animal-based ones.

Getting necessary nutrients through supplements is also not the answer (with the exception of vitamin B_{12}), as not enough studies have been done on the absorption level of those vitamins and minerals in the human body, and the FDA does not test or approve most supplements on the market. The importance of high fiber in the diet also cannot be overstated. A healthy digestive tract can prevent large bowel (colorectal) cancer and other diseases. Genetic predisposition is not the full story; nutrition plays an important role in determining what diseases emerge. Although adopting a plant-based diet can seem difficult at first, the body quickly gets accustomed to craving whole foods.

Key Terms

amino acids   the building blocks of **proteins**, they are necessary for many bodily functions. There are over one hundred amino acids found in nature, but only twenty are used by humans to synthesize the proteins required to sustain life. These twenty amino acids are classified as either "essential" or "nonessential." The nonessential amino acids are synthesized by the body, while the essential amino acids must be obtained from food.

antioxidant   a molecule that inhibits the process of oxidation in cells. Oxidation occurs when electrons from one molecule transfer to an oxidizing agent (basically, a molecule that allows a bond with an oxygen molecule). These reactions can cause the formation of **free radicals**, which in turn can cause cascading events that form negative chain reactions in a cell. When cellular damage occurs, it can cause the death of the cell, or promote the uninhibited growth of the cell (cancer). Antioxidants terminate these chain reactions by binding with and removing free radicals from the mix. Good examples of excellent sources of antioxidants include legumes such as small red beans and pinto beans, cranberries, blueberries, blackberries, prunes, raspberries, and artichokes.

ATP (adenosine triphosphate)   a coenzyme (meaning that it is used in concert with other enzymes) that is used as a chemical energy carrier in the cells of all known organisms. ATP is produced in the body through a variety of processes, but the most prevalent is called the "citric acid cycle" or Krebs cycle, wherein the enzyme adenosine is "phosphorylated" (phosphates are bound to the adenosine). When chemical energy is required, the bonds attaching the phosphates to the adenosine are broken, thus releasing the energy needed for cellular metabolism. When these bonds are broken, there is the concurrent release of metabolic byproducts, the most harmful of which are **free radicals**.

biomarker a molecule, gene, or characteristic by which a particular disease, pathological process, or physiological progression can be identified. Biomarkers can be used to identify the presence of many diseases as well as measure the severity or progression of the disease process. They have biological properties that can be identified and measured in bodily fluids or tissues. For instance, blood pressure is used as a tool to assess the risk of stroke. Cholesterol levels are used to gauge the threat for heart disease. Biomarkers can also be used to identify a particular disease state; for example, antibodies indicate the presence of infection, past or present. Additionally, a biomarker can be a substance that is introduced into the body in order to detect or diagnose a particular disease, such as when radioactive iodine is used to identify abnormalities in the thyroid gland.

carbohydrate any organic molecule consisting of carbon, hydrogen, and oxygen, usually found with a ratio of 1:2:1 (for instance, the chemical formula for glucose is $C_6H_{12}O_6$). Examples of carbohydrates include sugars, starches, cellulose, and gum. Carbohydrates fall into many classifications, depending on their size and structure, and are named for the number of simple sugars (monosaccharides) that are bonded together. For example, a grouping composed of more than ten simple sugars is called a polysaccharide. Carbohydrates are produced in plants via the process of photosynthesis and serve as the major source of energy in animal diets. They can also function as structural components in plants (cellulose is used to form cellular walls and, most importantly, is the source of fiber found in plant products).

carotenoid   pigmented (colored) molecules, usually yellow, orange, or red, that are found in plants. They assist with the process of photosynthesis, helping to produce the energy a plant needs to grow. There are over six hundred identified carotenoids. They are an important part of the diets of humans (and other animals) because they act as **antioxidants**. Colorful fruits and vegetables owe their hues to carotenoids, which is why nutritionists urge consumers to include a wide selection of brightly colored produce in their diet. Some carotenoids are good sources of vitamin A, which is vital for eye health. Most carotenoid-rich fruits and vegetables are also quite low in fat, with the notable exceptions of avocados and *gac* fruit (found mostly in southern China and Vietnam).

cholesterol   a fat-like white crystalline substance found in animal tissue that is important as a structural component of cellular membranes as well as in the synthesis of various steroid hormones such as estrogen, testosterone, and cortisol (the "stress hormone"). It is also used by the body to produce myelin, the substance that acts as insulation around the nerves, and helps with the production of bile (used by the digestive system to break down fats). It is produced by the liver or absorbed from food in the intestines. High levels of blood cholesterol are associated with a higher risk for heart disease, stroke, and gallstones.

free radicals   a metabolic byproduct of the cellular production of **ATP** (among other things), a free radical is an atom or molecule that has not formed all the chemical bonds available for attachment with other atoms. For example, H_2O, the water molecule, is composed of three atoms—two hydrogen atoms connected to one oxygen atom. Oxygen can form two bonds, whereas hydrogen can form only one bond. When only one hydrogen atom has bonded with an oxygen atom, this leaves one more oxygen bond available, and the one hydrogen–one oxygen unit is called a free radical because it has a "free" bond. This happens countless times during the normal metabolic processes, but it can become a problem if too many free radicals are produced and bond with molecules that they are not meant to bond with, causing unhealthful effects such as cellular damage, which can lead to cancers, metabolic diseases, and brain damage or dementia.

lipid   a naturally occurring fatty or waxy compound that is not water-soluble. Examples of lipids are waxes, oils, triglycerides (fats), and cholesterol. Although all fats are lipids, not all lipids are fats. Therefore, the terms *lipid* and *fat* cannot be used interchangeably. Major biological functions of lipids involve energy storage (in the form of fats) and cell signaling (the transfer of certain chemicals from one cell to another), and they are a primary structural component of cell membranes. Vitamins A, D, E, and K are considered lipids.

macronutrients   in humans, nutrients that are used in relatively large amounts: **proteins**, **carbohydrates**, and fats. Macronutrients provide energy to the body in the form of calories.

micronutrients   in humans, nutrients that are required in minute or small amounts, such as vitamins and minerals. Micronutrients are available with a varied and healthful eating regimen, and supplements are rarely required when a person consumes a nutritionally balanced diet.

protein   a molecule composed of chains of **amino acids**. The type and sequence of the amino acids are determined by the DNA of the cell that produces the protein. Proteins have several different functions: serving as structural material (keratin), as enzymes, as transporters (hemoglobin), as antibodies, as regulators of gene expression, and as cellular receptors that bind with various chemicals and other molecules. Protein that is consumed via the diet is broken down by the body into its component amino acids, which are then "restrung" into new proteins that the body requires.

veganism   a diet that contains no animal products. It can also be defined as a way of life in which no animal products are used. Vegans consume a diet consisting of plant-based whole foods, unrefined grains, nuts, seeds, legumes, fruits, and vegetables. A balanced vegan diet provides all the essential nutritional components required by the human body except vitamin B_{12}, which may have to be taken in supplement form.

Recommended Reading

T. Colin Campbell and Thomas M. Campbell II's ***The China Study: The Most Comprehensive Study of Nutrition Ever Conducted and the Startling Implications for Diet, Weight Loss, and Long-Term Health*** (BenBella Books, 2005) is one of America's best-selling books about nutrition. This examination of the correlations between the consumption of animal products and a variety of chronic, often fatal, diseases produces extremely compelling arguments for diets composed of unprocessed, plant-based foods. The research is both observational and laboratory-based, and has been ongoing for decades. The findings show that eating a plant-based diet that contains a low percentage of protein can lead to a reduction of the rates of various cancers, heart disease, and diabetes, as well as a variety of other diseases.

The following books provide reading related to the subjects covered in *The China Study*. This recommended reading covers more of the nutritional data and includes books that discuss plant-based diets as well.

Neal Barnard, MD, *Food for Life: How the New Four Food Groups Can Save Your Life* (Harmony, 1993)

Barnard has redefined the four food groups from meat, dairy, grains, and fruit and vegetables; he suggests that the four new groups should be grains, legumes, vegetables, and fruit. He shows how a diet high in these foods can radically decrease the chance of developing cancer and heart disease while drastically increasing life expectancy.

T. Colin Campbell, PhD, and Howard Jacobson, PhD, *Whole: Rethinking the Science of Nutrition* (BenBella Books, 2013)

Based on cutting-edge nutritional science, this book explains why whole foods and plant-based diets are far more healthful and disease-preventing than the traditional Western animal-based diet. In this follow-up to his best-selling book, *The China Study*, Campbell clarifies the whys and hows regarding nutrition and the disease processes that plague Americans today, and shows how whole foods derived from plant sources affect people at both the microscopic and macroscopic level.

Brenda Davis, RD, and Vesanto Melina, MS, RD, *Becoming Vegan: The Complete Guide to Adopting a Healthy Plant-Based Diet* (Book Publishing Company, 2000)

As more people become motivated to consume a vegan diet, either for health or ethical reasons, there is a lot of confusion surrounding what a vegan diet actually is. The authors explain what nutrients are necessary for survival and clarify what foods need to be consumed to ensure that all nutritional needs are met. They delineate what the needs are for various segments of the population, including infants, children, seniors, and pregnant women, as well as provide information on various eating disorders and how a vegan diet can help correct them.

Caldwell B. Esselstyn Jr., MD, *Prevent and Reverse Heart Disease: The Revolutionary, Scientifically Proven, Nutrition-Based Cure* (Avery Trade, 2008)

After over twenty years of study and research, Esselstyn has shown that a plant-based, oil-free diet can not only slow the progression of the disease but actually reverse it. As he explains the science behind his eating plan, he tells of people who have come to him over the years stating that they had been told that they had less than one year to live. Included are testimonials from some of these people, most of whom changed their diet and lifestyle and are still alive today.

Rip Esselstyn, *The Engine 2 Diet: The Texas Firefighter's 28-Day Save-Your-Life Plan that Lowers Cholesterol and Burns Away the Pounds* (Grand Central Life & Style, 2009)

When Rip Esselstyn, son of physician and nutritional researcher Caldwell Esselstyn Jr., MD, found that many of his fellow firefighters had dangerously high cholesterol, he used his experience with plant-based diets to create a healthful and lifesaving eating plan for them that includes whole grains, fresh fruit, vegetables, legumes, nuts, and seeds. This book covers the science behind the nutrition, contains dozens of recipes, and gives tips about how to properly stock your pantry.

Dean Ornish, MD, *The Spectrum: A Scientifically Proven Program to Feel Better, Live Longer, Lose Weight, and Gain Health*, revised edition (Ballantine Books, 2008)

Ornish, best-selling author of *Dr. Dean Ornish's Program for Reversing Heart Disease* and *Eat More, Weigh Less*, among many other books, wrote this one to show how people can customize healthful eating and living based on their needs, desires, and genetic predispositions. He lays out a diet and lifestyle that can prevent or reverse disease processes and even prolong life. The book also contains recipes from chef Art Smith that incorporate whole foods from plant sources.

John Robbins, *The Food Revolution: How Your Diet Can Save Your Life and Our World*, 10th anniversary edition, with a foreword by Dean Ornish, MD (Conari Press, 2010)

First published in 2001, *The Food Revolution* advocates against the consumption of genetically modified organisms (GMOs) and animal products of all kinds, including fish. Robbins writes about the dangers of the factory farming system and urges that diets be composed of plant-based ingredients obtained from local farms (thus avoiding fuel consumption and pollution while at the same time supporting neighbors) that offer products grown organically.

Gene Stone, ed., *Forks Over Knives: The Plant-Based Way to Health*, with a foreword by T. Colin Campbell, PhD, and Caldwell B. Esselstyn Jr., MD (The Experiment, 2011)

This book follows a film documentary of the same name, with the title implying that nutrition (forks) is a far better way to prevent or treat disease than modern medicine (knives, or scalpels). It includes the basic information included in the film regarding the benefits of eating a whole-food, plant-based diet as well as insights from the scientists featured, success stories from people who have converted to a plant-based diet, tips on transitioning from an animal-based diet, and a recipe section.

Bibliography

Wilfred Niels Arnold, "The China Study"

Leonardo, last modified February 1, 2005

http://www.leonardo.info/reviews/feb2005/china_arnold.html

Independent Science News. **Unsigned review of** *The China Study: The Most Comprehensive Study of Nutrition Ever Conducted and the Startling Implications for Diet, Weight Loss, and Long-Term Health,* **by T. Collin Campbell, PhD, and Thomas M. Campbell II, MD**

February 6, 2010

http://independentsciencenews.org/health/the-china-study

David S. Martin, "From Omnivore to Vegan: The Dietary Education of Bill Clinton"

CNN, August 18, 2011

http://www.cnn.com/2011/HEALTH/08/18/bill.clinton.diet.vegan/index.html

Denise Minger, "The China Study: Fact or Fallacy?"

Raw Food SOS (blog), July 7, 2010

http://rawfoodsos.com/2010/07/07/the-china-study-fact-or-fallac

Lawrence Wilson, MD, "The China Study, a False Book"

DrLWilson.com, 2013

http://drlwilson.com/Articles/CHINA%20STUDY%20BOOK%20REVIEW.htm

Lightning Source UK Ltd.
Milton Keynes UK
UKOW05f2142050813

214918UK00002B/344/P